Contents

What Is a Low-Sodium Diet?

A low sodium diet is a diet that is low in salt, usually allowing less than 1 teaspoon per day. Many diseases, including kidney disease, heart disease, and diabetes, require a patient to follow a low sodium diet.

The Role of Sodium

The majority of sodium consumed comes from sodium chloride (NaCl), better known as salt. Salt has many useful properties, both in food preservation and for the body. It helps to prevent spoilage by drawing the moisture out of foods. This helps to keep bacteria from growing in the food. It can also kill bacteria that are already growing on the surface of foods. Before refrigeration technology was developed, salting was one of the few methods available for preserving foods, such as meat, through the winter. Salt also dissolves into the electrolytes Na+ and Cl1 that help maintain the right balance of fluids in the body, transmit signals through the nervous system, and cause muscles to contract and relax.

The kidneys are responsible for regulating the amount of sodium in the body. When the body has too much sodium, the kidneys filter some out and the excess amounts are excreted from the body in the urine. When the body does not have enough sodium, the kidneys help to conserve sodium and return the needed amount into the bloodstream. When a person eats too much salt, however, and the kidneys are not able to filter enough out, sodium begins to build up in the blood. In the same way that salt pulls water out of foods, sodium in the blood pulls out and holds water from cells in the body. This increases the volume of the blood and puts strain on the heart and circulatory system.

Ways to Reduce Salt Intake

According to a study done by the Mayo Clinic, the average American gets only 6% of their total salt intake from salt that is added at the table. Only 5% comes from salt that is added during cooking, and natural sources in food makeup only another 11 percent. The remaining 77% comes from processed or prepared foods. Many packaged meats, as well as canned and frozen foods, contain a surprising amount of salt. Salt is used so heavily by manufacturers because it acts as a preservative, adds flavor to foods, helps to keep foods from drying out, and can even increase the sweetness in desserts. Soups are often especially high in salt because salt helps to disguise chemical or metallic aftertaste.

One of the best ways to reduce salt intake is to cut back on heavily processed and prepared foods. Hot dogs, sausages, ham, and prepackaged deli meats usually contain much more salt than freshly sliced lean meats, such as chicken or fish. Most canned vegetables also have a much higher salt content than the same vegetable found in the fresh produce section. Frozen prepared meals should be avoided for the same reason, and canned soups usually contain much more salt than soups made a home. By reading the Nutrition Facts label on the side of commercially manufactured foods, dieters can determine how much sodium is in the food they are considering.

When choosing canned or frozen foods, dieters who wish to reduce their salt intake can often find a 'low sodium' option. The Food and Drug Administration (FDA) sets legal standards for how much sodium can be contained in a product that is labeled 'low sodium.' Products labeled as such may not contain more than 140 milligrams of sodium per serving, while products labeled as 'reduced sodium' need only contain 25% less sodium than the usual amount found in that product.

Meals served in restaurants are also often high in salt. Most restaurant kitchens use a great deal of processed foods. To this they often add salt because it is an inexpensive way to improve the taste. Recently, some chain restaurants have begun providing dietary information about their meals. Usually this is printed in a pamphlet that is separate from the menu, so customers may need to ask for it. Some restaurant chains even provide this information on their websites so that customers can decide on a low-sodium meal before they visit the restaurant. If this information is not available, dieters can use the same ideas for avoiding salt at the restaurant that they do at the supermarket. Salads and other foods made with fresh vegetables will usually have less salt than soups. Appetizers and meals with sauces should generally be avoided.

Another time that salt can be eliminated from the diet is when cooking or preparing meals at home. With the exception of baked goods, many recipes that call for salt do so only for taste, and it can be left out. By substituting herbs and spices for salt, the cook can avoid making bland food while still avoiding salt. When choosing an herb or spice mixture, it is important that the dieter select one that is not itself high in sodium. Using the zest of a lemon or lime is another a good way to add flavor without adding salt. There are also artificial salt substitutes available, although kidney patients should avoid these as they are usually high in potassium, another mineral that is regulated by the kidneys.

The most obvious way to reduce salt intake is to cut back on the amount of salt added at the table. Since salt is an acquired taste, many doctors recommend simply removing the salt shaker from the table altogether. Most condiments like ketchup, mustard, and pickle relish are also high in salt. Eliminating these can also be a significant help. Many commercially available sauces, dips, and salad dressings also contain a lot of salt. By checking the labels on these condiments before purchasing, consumers can often find options with less sodium.

Sodium Content of Popular Foods

Many people are unaware of just how much sodium is in some of the most popular foods. A low sodium diet generally consists of 1500 to

2400 milligrams of sodium each day. Some foods contain almost half of this in a single serving. The following is a list of foods and the approximate amount of sodium in one serving of each of them.

- 1 large cheeseburger: 1,220 mg

- 1 cup canned soup: 800 mg

- 1 hot dog: 650 mg

- 12-ounce can of soda: 25 mg

- 1/2 cup cottage cheese: 425 mg

- 1 Tablespoon soy sauce: 800 mg

- 1 bean burrito: 920 mg

- 1 Saltine cracker: 70 mg

- 1 frozen enchilada: 680 mg

Function

The low sodium diet is designed to lower the amount of sodium that a person consumes. While this is generally considered healthy for most Americans, a low sodium diet is particularly important for people suffering from certain conditions and diseases.

For kidney patients, reducing sodium is important because the kidneys are no longer capable of effectively filtering sodium out of the body. If these patients do not reduce their sodium intake, the buildup of sodium will cause fluid retention, which can cause swelling in the lower extremities. A low sodium diet will help to prevent this problem. For heart patients, a low sodium diet is important to help reduce strain on the heart. Excess sodium in the bloodstream means that excess fluid is kept suspended, which increases the volume that the heart must pump.

Benefits

There are benefits of a low sodium diet for people suffering from many different diseases and even for those who are not. A diet that is low in sodium can help to reduce blood pressure and the risk of heart disease and stroke. People who have a family history of heart problems, people of African decent, smokers, those who frequently drink alcohol, people who are overweight or do not exercise regularly, and people who live with a lot of unmanaged stress are all at higher risk for increase blood pressure and should consider a low sodium diet. For heart disease patients, a low sodium diet can be part of a plan to reduce their blood pressure and reduce the strain on their heart in order to slow the progress of current conditions and prevent future problems. For kidney patients, a low sodium diet is necessary to prevent fluid retention.

Precautions

Anyone thinking of significantly altering their regular diet should talk to their physician. Each person has different dietary needs, which should be considered. In general, moderately lowering sodium intake is considered safe for most people. Dieters should be careful to not severely and abruptly increase their level of exercise and fluid intake while severely and abruptly lowering their sodium intake to avoid hyponatremia.

Risks

The risks of following a low sodium diet are very low. Many experts believe that most Americans could benefit from following a low sodium diet, even if they do not yet suffer from any of the conditions that might require them to do so. Most Americans consume between 3000 and 5000 milligrams of sodium per day, and a low sodium diet reduces this to a healthier level of between 1500 and 2400 milligrams per day. Since the physiological requirement for sodium for adults is only 500 milligrams daily, there is little danger that a person following a low sodium diet will consume so little sodium that it will endanger their health.

Some athletes and others who exercise frequently and ingest very little sodium yet drink a lot of water may be at risk of hyponatremia, a condition that occurs when the body does not have enough sodium. Though rare, low sodium levels can cause headache, nausea, lethargy, confusion, muscle twitching, and convulsions.

QUESTIONS TO ASK THE DOCTOR

- What kinds of foods should I avoid?

- How much sodium is best for me?

- Which foods are low in sodium?

- How will I know if I am consuming too little sodium?

- Are there any sign or symptoms that might indicate a problem while on this diet?

What Foods Are Highest in Sodium?

Foods highest in sodium are table salt, fast foods, preserved foods, and processed foods, such as:

- Canned foods

- Frozen dinners

- Snack food

- Packaged starchy foods—like seasoned rice, instant mashed potatoes, macaroni and cheese

- Baking mixes

- Deli meats and cheeses

• Sausages and cured or smoked meats

Food Choices on a Low-Sodium Diet

Grains

Foods you can eat are:

• Breads and rolls without salted tops

• Ready-to-eat and uncooked cereals (with less than 5% Daily Value [DV] for sodium)

• Muffins

• Unsalted crackers and breadsticks

• Low-sodium or homemade breadcrumbs or stuffing

• Rice, pasta, bulgur, couscous (made without salt)

Foods you should not eat are:

- Breads, rolls, and crackers with salted tops

- Quick breads, self-rising flour, and biscuit mixes

- Regular bread crumbs

- Instant hot cereals

- Commercially made rice, pasta, or stuffing mixes

Veggies

Foods you should eat are:

- All fresh veggies

- Frozen and canned veggies without added salt

- Low-sodium vegetable juices

Foods you should not eat are:

- Regular canned veggies and juices

- Sauerkraut

- Frozen veggies with sauces

- Commercially made potato and veggie mixes

Fruits

Foods you should eat are:

- Fresh, frozen, and canned juices

- Fruit juices

Foods you should not eat are:

- None

Dairy

Foods you should eat are:

- Milk

- Yogurt

- Hard cheeses, such as Swiss, cheddar, and Monterey Jack

- Low-sodium cheeses, such as ricotta, cream cheese, and mozzarella

- Ice cream

Foods you should not eat are:

- Processed cheese, cottage cheese, cheese spreads, and sauces

- Buttermilk

Meats and Beans

Foods you should eat are:

- Fresh or frozen beef, lamb, pork, poultry, fish, and shellfish

- Eggs and egg substitutes

- Low-sodium peanut butter

- Dried peas and beans

- Unsalted nuts

Foods you should not eat are:

- Smoked, cured, salted, or canned meat, fish, or poultry—including bacon, cold cuts, frankfurters, sausages, sardines, and anchovies

- Frozen, breaded meats

- Salted nuts

Fats and Oils

Foods you should eat are:

- Low-sodium or unsalted butter and margarine spreads

- Low-sodium salad dressings made with oil

Foods you should not eat are:

• Oil mixed with other, high-sodium items—like prepared salad dressings

Snacks, Sweets, and Condiments

Foods you can eat are:

• Low-sodium or unsalted versions of broths, soups, soy sauce, condiments, and snack foods

• Pepper, herbs, spices, vinegar, lemon, or lime juice

• Ice cream, sherbet, homemade pie, and pudding without added salt

Foods you should not eat are:

• Broth, soups, gravies, and sauces made from instant mixes or other high-sodium items

• Salted snack foods

- Olives

- Meat tenderizers, seasoning salt, and most flavored vinegars

- Commercial dessert mixes, cake, pie, instant pudding

Drinks

Drinks you can have are:

- Most drinks

Drinks you should not have are:

- Commercially softened water

Tips

- Eat plenty of whole grains, fruits, and veggies. Choose whole foods over processed foods.

- Read food labels. Look for products marked as:

- Sodium-free

- Very low-sodium

- Low-sodium

- No added salt

- Unsalted

- Skip the salt when cooking or at the table. Use herbs, spices, garlic, and onion to add flavor to foods.

- Do not eat fast foods. They have a lot of added salt.

- Talk to a dietitian for help with meal planning.

Low-Sodium Diet Plan: 1,500 Calories

In this low-sodium diet plan, flavor-packed meals and snacks clock in under 1,500 mg of sodium per day.

Salt can quickly turn a bland dish into something delicious. A little bit goes a long way to amp up the flavor and it's definitely a kitchen essential. But the trouble with salt is that too much salt over time can contribute to conditions like hypertension (also known as high blood pressure), heart disease and kidney problems. Thankfully, there are simple ways you can cut down the salt in your diet (subsequently decreasing your risk for those related health conditions), without sacrificing flavor. In this low-sodium diet plan, we show you how to do just that with a week of flavor-packed meals and snacks that all clock in under 1,500 mg of sodium per day-the recommended amount to stay under when following a low-sodium diet.

While a heavy hand with the saltshaker can partly be to blame, packaged foods are really what puts us over the edge on sodium, as they tend to be high in salt for both flavor and preservation. In this meal plan, healthy low-sodium home-cooked recipes come together easily and use salt-free flavorings, like herbs and spices, to amp up the flavor while keeping the sodium in check. We also included plenty of high-potassium foods like bananas, avocados, cantaloupe and dark leafy greens, because potassium helps to cancel out the negative effects of sodium. This low-sodium diet plan makes it easy to eat healthy while keeping things as delicious as ever.

If you're looking for a meal plan that also controls for saturated fat, follow along with this Heart-Healthy Meal Plan at 1,500 Calories.

How to Meal Prep Your Week of Meals:

1. Make the Zucchini Noodles with Quick Turkey Bolognese and store in 4 separate meal-prep containers to have for lunch on Days 2, 3, 4 and 5.

2. Take some time each night to pack up your snacks for the next day ahead of time so they're ready to grab and go in the morning.

Day 1

Breakfast (354 calories, 157 mg sodium)

- 1 servingQuick-Cooking Oats

- 1/4 cup raisins

- 2 Tbsp. chopped walnuts

Top oats with raisins, walnuts and a pinch of cinnamon.

A.M. Snack (265 calories, 115 mg sodium)

- 1 cup frozen raspberries, thawed

- 1 cup whole-milk plain yogurt

- 2 tsp. honey

Lunch (396 calories, 466 mg sodium)

- 1 serving Quick Creamy Tomato Cup-of-Soup

- 1 medium orange

Easy Grilled Cheese

- 1 Tbsp. unsalted butter

- 1 slice whole-wheat bread, halved

- 2 Tbsp. shredded Cheddar cheese

Spread butter on one side of each bread half. Place 1 slice, buttered-side down, in a warm skillet. Top with cheese and the other slice of bread, buttered-side up. Cook on each side until golden brown and the cheese has melted.

P.M. Snack (82 calories, 38 mg sodium)

- 1 1/2 cups cubed cantaloupe

Dinner (428 calories, 706 mg sodium)

- 1 serving Philly Cheesesteak Stuffed Peppers

- 1 1/2 servings Steak Fries (about 9 wedges)

Daily Totals: 1,525 calories, 65 g protein, 196 g carbohydrate, 31 g fiber, 63 g fat, 26 g saturated fat, 3,697 mg potassium, 1,482 mg sodium

Day 2

Breakfast (357 calories, 238 mg sodium)

• 1 serving Spinach-Avocado Smoothie

A.M. Snack (318 calories, 114 mg sodium)

• 1 cup frozen raspberries, thawed

• 1 cup whole-milk plain yogurt

• 2 Tbsp. chopped walnuts

Lunch (336 calories, 555 mg sodium)

- 1 serving Zucchini Noodles with Quick Turkey Bolognese topped with 1 Tbsp. basil-infused olive oil

P.M. Snack (54 calories, 26 mg sodium)

- 1 cup cubed cantaloupe

Dinner (430 calories, 586 mg sodium)

- 1 serving Easy Pea & Spinach Carbonara

Daily Totals: 1,495 calories, 70 g protein, 171 g carbohydrate, 31 g fiber, 66 g fat, 17 g saturated fat, 3,529 mg potassium, 1,520 mg sodium

Day 3

Breakfast (440 calories, 406 mg sodium)

- 1 serving Peanut Butter & Chia Berry Jam English Muffin

- 1/2 serving Spinach-Avocado Smoothie

Meal-Prep Tip: Save the other 1/2 serving of the Spinach-Avocado Smoothie to have on Day 5.

A.M. Snack (54 calories, 26 mg sodium)

- 1 cup cubed cantaloupe

Lunch (336 calories, 555 mg sodium)

- 1 serving Zucchini Noodles with Quick Turkey Bolognese topped with 1 Tbsp. basil-infused olive oil

P.M. Snack (210 calories, 54 mg sodium)

- 1 medium banana
- 1 Tbsp. peanut butter

Dinner (374 calories, 378 mg sodium)

• 1 serving Skillet Lemon Chicken & Potatoes with Kale

Evening Snack (93 calories, 2 mg sodium)

• 3 cups air-popped popcorn topped with 1 Tbsp. no-salt-added garlic & herb seasoning

Related: How to Make DIY Popcorn 4 Ways

Daily Totals: 1,508 calories, 71 g protein, 172 g carbohydrate, 29 g fiber, 67 g fat, 13 g saturated fat, 3,638 mg potassium, 1,420 mg sodium

Day 4

Breakfast (357 calories, 238 mg sodium)

- 1 serving Spinach-Avocado Smoothie

A.M. Snack (64 calories, 1 mg sodium)

- 1 cup raspberries

Lunch (336 calories, 555 mg sodium)

- 1 serving Zucchini Noodles with Quick Turkey Bolognese topped with 1 Tbsp. basil-infused olive oil

P.M. Snack (210 calories, 54 mg sodium)

- 1 medium banana

- 1 Tbsp. peanut butter

Dinner (484 calories, 228 mg sodium)

- 1 serving Salmon with Cilantro-Pineapple Salsa

- 1 cup Easy Brown Rice

Evening Snack (62 calories, 1 mg sodium)

- 2 cups air-popped popcorn topped with 1 Tbsp. no-salt-added garlic & herb seasoning

Daily Totals: 1,513 calories, 73 g protein, 191 g carbohydrate, 30 g fiber, 57 g fat, 11 g saturated fat, 3,811 mg potassium, 1,077 mg sodium

Day 5

Meal-Prep Tip: The Pork Carnitas recipe for tonight's dinner is a slow-cooker recipe. Get it going early enough in the day so it's ready come dinnertime.

Breakfast (440 calories, 406 mg sodium)

- 1 serving Peanut Butter & Chia Berry Jam English Muffin

- 1/2 serving Spinach-Avocado Smoothie

A.M. Snack (109 calories, 51 mg sodium)

- 2 cups cubed cantaloupe

Lunch (296 calories, 555 mg sodium)

- 1 serving Zucchini Noodles with Quick Turkey Bolognese topped with 2 tsp. basil-infused olive oil

P.M. Snack (64 calories, 1 mg sodium)

- 1 cup raspberries

Dinner (549 calories, 480 mg sodium)

- 1 servingPork Carnitas(2 tacos)

- 2 Tbsp. reduced-fat sour cream

- 2 Tbsp. diced tomatoes

Top tacos with sour cream and tomatoes. For a spicy kick, sprinkle on a no-salt-added spice like cayenne pepper or crushed red pepper.

- 1 serving Pineapple & Avocado Salad

Meal-Prep Tip: Save 1/2 serving of the Pork Carnitas (1 taco) and 1 serving of the Pineapple & Avocado Salad to have for lunch on Day 6.

Evening Snack (62 calories, 0 mg sodium)

- medium orange

Daily Totals: 1,520 calories, 78 g protein, 187 g carbohydrate, 40 g fiber, 61 g fat, 14 g saturated fat, 3,656 mg potassium, 1,493 mg sodium

Day 6

Breakfast (440 calories, 406 mg sodium)

• 1 serving Peanut Butter & Chia Berry Jam English Muffin • 1/2 serving Spinach-Avocado Smoothie

Meal-Prep Tip: Save the other 1/2 serving of the Spinach-Avocado Smoothie to have on Day 7.

A.M. Snack (185 calories, 86 mg sodium)

• 1 cup frozen raspberries, thawed

• 3/4 cup whole-milk plain yogurt

Lunch (349 calories, 264 mg sodium)

• 1/2 serving Pork Carnitas (1 taco)

• 2 Tbsp. diced tomatoes

Top taco with tomatoes. For a spicy kick, sprinkle on a no-salt-added spice like cayenne pepper or crushed red pepper.

- 1 serving Pineapple & Avocado Salad

P.M. Snack (109 calories, 51 mg sodium)

- 2 cups cubed cantaloupe

Dinner (346 calories, 665 mg sodium)

- 1 serving Shrimp Scampi Zoodles

- 1 (1-inch-thick) slice whole-wheat baguette, toasted

Evening Snack (62 calories, 0 mg sodium)

- 1 medium orange

Daily Totals: 1,491 calories, 78 g protein, 190 g carbohydrate, 38 g fiber, 55 g fat, 16 g saturated fat, 3,804 mg potassium, 1,473 mg sodium

Day 7

Breakfast (307 calories, 157 mg sodium)

• 1 servingQuick-Cooking Oats

• 1/4 cup raisins

• 1 Tbsp. chopped walnuts

Top oats with raisins, walnuts and a pinch of cinnamon.

A.M. Snack (243 calories, 120 mg sodium)

• 1/2 serving Spinach-Avocado Smoothie • 1 cup raspberries

Lunch (301 calories, 466 mg sodium)

- 1 serving Quick Creamy Tomato Cup-of-Soup

Easy Grilled Cheese

- 2 tsp. unsalted butter

- 1 slice whole-wheat bread, halved

- 2 Tbsp. shredded Cheddar cheese

Spread butter on one side of the bread slices. Place 1 slice, buttered-side down, in a warm skillet. Top with cheese and the other slice of bread, buttered-side up. Cook on each side until golden brown and the cheese has melted.

P.M. Snack (210 calories, 54 mg sodium)

- 1 medium banana

- 1 Tbsp. peanut butter

Dinner (465 calories, 359 mg sodium)

- 1 serving Jerk Chicken & Pineapple Slaw

- 1 cup Easy Brown Rice

Daily Totals: 1,525 calories, 66 g protein, 227 g carbohydrate, 32 g fiber, 46 g fat, 13 g saturated fat, 3,683 mg potassium, 1,155 mg sodium

LOW SODIUM DIET RECIPES

Trying new low sodium-friendly recipes is a great way to explore new flavors and find new favorite dishes while looking after your health. In this part are nourishing low sodium diet recipes for you to enjoy.

Low sodium Tacos

Preparation time

35 minutes

Ingredients

- 2 pounds lean ground beef

- Hard-shell tacos

Taco Toppings

- 1 head of lettuce, shredded

- 2 Roma tomatoes, diced

- 1 medium white onion, diced

- 1/2 cup sour cream

Taco Seasoning

- 3 tablespoons chili powder

- 1 tablespoon ground cumin

- 3/4 teaspoon onion powder

- 3/4 teaspoon garlic powder

Instructions

1. In a small bowl, mix taco seasoning until blended.

2. In a large skillet over medium-high heat, brown meat, and stir in seasoning.

3. Fill the taco shell with meat, tomatoes, 1 tablespoon of chopped onion, lettuce, and add a dollop of sour cream.

Blackened Chicken with Avocado Cream Sauce

Preparation time

25 minutes

Ingredients

- 4 (4-ounce) boneless, skinless chicken breasts

- 2 tablespoons blackened seasoning

- ½ cup plain, 0% Greek yogurt

- ½ avocado

- 1 teaspoon lemon juice

- ½ teaspoon garlic powder

- ⅛ teaspoon salt

- 2 tablespoons green onions, thinly sliced

Instructions

1. Place the chicken breasts and blackened seasoning in a large resealable bag.

2. Seal and shake a few times to evenly coat the chicken.

3. Lightly coat a large skillet with nonstick cooking spray and heat over medium-high heat. Add the chicken and cook until cooked through, 4 to 6 minutes per side.

4. Meanwhile, in a food processor, combine the yogurt, avocado, lemon juice, garlic powder, and salt and pulse until smooth and creamy.

5. To serve, top each chicken breast with 2 tablespoons of the creamy avocado sauce and garnish with ½ tablespoon green onions.

SIMPLE SESAME CHICKEN

Preparation time

35 minutes

INGREDIENTS

- 2 pounds boneless, skinless chicken breasts, cut into pieces

- 1/2 teaspoon salt

- 1/2 teaspoons pepper

- 3 tablespoons flour

- 2 tablespoons toasted sesame oil

- 1 tablespoon olive oil

- 2 garlic cloves, minced

- 1 tablespoon low-sodium soy sauce

- 1 tablespoon brown sugar

- 1 tablespoon white vinegar

- 1/2 cup low-sodium chicken stock

- 2-3 tablespoons toasted sesame seeds

• brown rice and vegetables for serving

INSTRUCTIONS

1. Preheat oven to 400 degrees F.

2. In a bowl, whisk together chicken stock, brown sugar, 1 tablespoon sesame oil, garlic cloves, soy sauce and vinegar. Set aside.

3. Heat a large oven-proof skillet over medium-high heat.

4. Toss chicken with salt, pepper and flour.

5. Add olive oil and 1 tablespoon sesame oil to skillet, and once hot, add chicken in a single layer.

6. Cook until seared and golden on one side, then flip and cook until golden again, about 2-3 minutes.

7. Pour chicken stock mixture over top and toss to coat, then turn off heat.

8. Place skillet in oven and bake for 20 minutes.

9. Remove and cover with sesame seeds.

10. Serve with veggie of your choice and brown rice.

Light and Easy Pasta Primavera

Preparation time

35 minutes

Ingredients

- 8 ounces gemelli pasta, dry

- 2 cups broccoli florets

- ½ cup matchstick carrots

- 1 red bell pepper, thinly sliced

- 1½ tablespoons extra virgin olive oil

- ½ onion, thinly sliced

- 1 tablespoon minced garlic

- 1 small zucchini, thinly sliced in half moons (about 1½ cups)

- 1 small yellow squash, thinly sliced in half moons (about 1½ cups)

- ½ cup cherry tomatoes, halved

- ½ cup frozen peas

- ½ cup white cooking wine

- juice of ½ lemon (about 1 tablespoon) + ½ teaspoon zest

- ⅓ cup reduced-fat grated Parmesan cheese

- 2 tablespoons fresh parsley, chopped

Instructions

1. Bring a large pot of salted water to a boil, and cook the pasta according to package directions for al dente.

2. Remove with a slotted spoon, and reserve in a bowl.

3. Do not drain the pasta water.

4. Bring the water back up to a boil and cook the broccoli, carrots, and bell pepper slices until they are bright and tender crisp, 2 minutes.

5. Drain the vegetables and set aside.

6. Heat a large skillet over medium heat and add the oil, onions, and garlic.

7. Cook until the onions are soft, 4-6 minutes.

8. Add the zucchini, yellow squash, and tomatoes and continue cooking until they begin to soften, 2-4 minutes.

9. Adjust the heat to medium-high and add the peas, the set-aside vegetables, the cooking wine, lemon juice, and lemon zest and simmer until the sauce slightly thickens, 3-4 minutes.

10. Reduce the heat to low and add the set-aside cooked pasta, the cheese, and parsley to the skillet.

11. Toss gently with tongs to evenly coat all the ingredients in the sauce, and serve hot.

5 -INGREDIENT BUTTERNUT SQUASH, ARUGULA AND GOAT CHEESE PASTA

Preparation time

40 minutes

INGREDIENTS

• 1 medium butternut squash, peeled, seeded and diced into 3/4-inch cubes

• 1 tablespoon vegetable oil (or any high-heat oil)

• salt and freshly-cracked black pepper

• 12 ounces whole wheat dried pasta

- 2 ounces goat cheese

- 2 big handfuls fresh baby arugula

- 1/3 cup toasted pine nuts

INSTRUCTIONS

1. Heat oven to 425°F.

2. Line a baking sheet with parchment paper (or mist it with cooking spray).

3. In a large mixing bowl, combine the butternut squash and oil, and toss until the squash is evenly coated.

4. Spread the squash out the prepared baking sheet in an even layer.

5. Bake for 20-25 minutes, flipping the squash at the halfway point then returning them to the oven, until the squash are cooked through and soft on the inside.

6. Remove and set aside.

7. While the squash is cooking, bring a large stockpot of generously-salted water to a boil. Add the pasta and cook al dente, according to package instructions.

8. Once it reaches al dente, scoop out about 1 cup of the pasta water and set it aside for later.

9. Then drain the rest of the water and return the pasta to the stockpot.

10. Immediately add in the goat cheese along with 1/4 cup of the reserved pasta water, and toss until the cheese is completely melted and is

evenly coating the pasta. (If it seems too thick and you'd like a lighter "sauce", add in a few more tablespoons of the pasta water at a time until the cheese reaches your desired consistency.)

11. Add in the arugula, pine nuts and roasted butternut squash, and toss until combined.

12. Serve immediately, garnished with extra black pepper if desired.

Low Sodium Buffalo Wings

Preparation time

55 minutes

INGREDIENTS

- 24 Chicken Wings

- 3 T Unsalted Butter

- 3 T Tabasco Sauce or other Low Sodium Hot Sauce

- 2 T White Vinegar

- Cooking Spray to coat the foil on the roasting pan

INSTRUCTIONS

1. Thaw the wings to room temperature and pat them dry with a paper towelto remove any extra moisture

2. With cooking shears or a knife, cut off and discard the small tip of each wing.

3. Also cut the main wing bone and second wing bone at the joint.

4. Line a ¾" deep baking sheet with foil, and spray a light coating of cooking spray.

5. Place the wings on the sheet and bake in a 350 degree F oven until crisp, about 30-40 minutes.

6. Melt the butter in small saucepan over medium-high heat; and whisk in the hot sauce and vinegar.

7. Place wings in a large bowl or container that can be covered with a lid, or some foil.

8. Pour sauce over the wings, cover the bowl tightly with foil or a lid and shake to coat the wings.

9. Remove wings from the sauce and collect the remaining sauce in a bowl for guests who want more sauce.

Paleo taco salad

Preparation time

1 hour

INGREDIENTS

Creamy spicy dressing

- 2 ounces hemp seeds (1/2 cup) raw, soaked for at least 4 hours

- 2 tbsp olive oil (extra virgin)

- 2 tbsp water (filtered or spring)

- 1 tbsp white vinegar use lemon juice if not on the migraine diet

- 1 clove garlic

- 1/2 tsp white pepper

- 1/2 tsp smoked paprika (pimenton)

- 1/2 tsp cumin (dried)

- 1 sprig Italian flat-leaf parsley (fresh) or cilantro

- 4 small cherry tomatoes

- Taco seasoning

- 2 tbsp chili powder preferably California chili powder

- 2 tbsp smoked paprika (pimenton)

- 1 tbsp cumin (dried)

- 1 tbsp garlic powder

- 1 tbsp onion powder (omit for migraine diet)

- 1/2 tsp oregano (dried)

- 1/4 tsp chipotle powder or cayenne

Salad

- 16 ounces beef (grass-fed) ground (see above for vegan substitutes)

- 2 bell peppers (capsicum), red and yellow, thinly sliced

- 2 onions (green) scallions, spring onions, sliced on the diagonal

- 4 cups romaine lettuce salad greens, spring mix

- 1 pint cherry tomatoes

- 1 avocado

- 3 radishes thinly sliced, or jicama cut into sticks

INSTRUCTIONS

Creamy spicy dressing

1. Soak the hemp seeds in filtered water for at least four hours.

2. Drain and rinse thoroughly.

3. Place all dressing ingredients in the blender and blend until smooth and creamy. Set aside.

Taco seasoning

1. Mix all ingredients together until one color. This makes enough for two recipes.

Salad

1. Heat a cast-iron skillet over medium-high heat.

2. Add the beef, breaking up with a spoon and cooking until no longer pink.

3. Sprinkle 3 tbsp taco seasoning evenly over the beef and add one cup (200 ml) of filtered water. Stir to mix thoroughly.

4. Continue to cook over medium heat until the moisture is gone and beef is cooked.

5. Remove beef to a warm plate.

6. Do not wipe out the pan.

7. Add 1 tbsp (15 ml) coconut oil, extra-virgin olive oil, or rendered bacon fat to the pan, tilting to coat evenly.

8. Sauté the peppers and the green onion for 10 minutes until golden and fairly limp.

9. To serve as shown, lay out ingredients on a large platter with the dressing on the side.

Seared Flank Steak With Steamed Asparagus and Turnip-Sweet Potato Mash

Preparation time

10 hours

INGREDIENTS

For the steak (prepared this morning):

- 1 teaspoon canola oil

- 1 tablespoon tamari

- 1 clove crushed garlic

- 8 ounces flank steak, fat trimmed

- 1/2 tablespoon canola oil, to cook the steak\

For the turnip-sweet potato mash:

- 1 small sweet potato, peeled and cut in 1-inch cubes

- 2 medium turnips, peeled and cut in ½-inch cubes

- Kosher salt and freshly ground pepper

- 1 ounce soft goat cheese, crumbled

For the asparagus:

- 1 bunch asparagus, woody ends trimmed

Instructions

1. To marinate the steak (prepared this morning):

2. In a medium airtight container, stir together the canola oil, honey, tamari, and crushed garlic.

3. Add the skirt steak and coat it with the marinade. Marinate for 8 to 12 hours in the fridge.

For the turnip-sweet potato mash:

1. In the microwave: Put the sweet potato and turnips in a microwave-safe bowl with 2 tablespoons of water and a pinch of salt.

2. Cover and cook on high until the vegetables are very soft, 7 to 8 minutes.

3. On the stovetop: Put the sweet potato and turnips in a small pot with ½ cup water and a pinch of salt.

4. Bring the water to a boil, then reduce to a simmer, cover the pot, and cook until the vegetables are very soft, 12 to 15 minutes.

5. Drain the cooked vegetables, season with salt and pepper, and add the crumbled goat cheese.

6. Mash with two forks until the mixture is combined but lumpy.

For the steak:

1. Take the steak out of the marinade and pat it dry with paper towels.

2. Heat the canola oil in a medium skillet over medium-high heat.

3. Add the steak to the pan. For a steak that's about ½ inch thick, cook it 3 minutes, then flip and cook for another 2 minutes for medium-rare.

4. Cook an additional few minutes on each side for a more well-done steak.

5. Cook a thinner steak for a little less time and a thicker steak for a little more time.

6. Let the steak rest on a cutting board for at least 5 minutes, then cut it in half, against the grain.

7. Cut half the steak into thin slices.

8. For the asparagus: In a large skillet with a lid, bring ¼ cup water to a simmer with a pinch of kosher salt.

9. Add the asparagus to the skillet, turn the heat to low and simmer 4 to 5 minutes, until asparagus is cooked through but still slightly crunchy.

10. Serve the sliced half-steak, half the asparagus and half the vegetable mash for dinner.

11. Leftovers: Let the remaining halves of the steak, asparagus, and vegetable mash cool, then refrigerate them in separate airtight containers.

Crockpot Sweet Potato & Black Bean Quinoa Chili

Preparation time

30 minutes

Ingredients

- 3 cups diced sweet potato about 1 large

- 1 cup diced red onion about 1 medium

- 1 cup diced bell peppers about 1 large

- 3 garlic cloves minced

- 1 15 oz can organic black beans

- 1 28 oz can of fire roasted tomatoes

- 3 – 4 cups vegetable broth

- 2 tablespoons tomato paste

- 1/2 cup uncooked quinoa

- 1 – 1 1/2 tablespoons chili powder

- 2 teaspoons cumin

- 2 teaspoons paprika

- 1 teaspoon coriander

- 1/2 teaspoon cayenne more or less to taste

- Salt & pepper to taste

Instructions

1. Add all ingredients into a crock pot (starting with just 3 cups of broth).

2. Turn on high and cook for 4 hours, turn down to low and continue to cook until ready to serve. If too thick, stir in another ½ – 1 cup of water.

3. Serve with diced avocado (or guac) and tortilla chips. It's such a good combo!

ONE POT LEMON HERB CHICKEN & RICE

Preparation time

30 minutes

INGREDIENTS

• 4 boneless skinless chicken breasts

• 2 tablespoons butter

• salt and pepper to taste

• 2 teaspoons Italian seasoning

Rice

• 1 cup uncooked white rice

• 2 1/4 cups chicken broth (I used low sodium)

• juice of 1 lemon

• 1 teaspoon Italian seasoning

INSTRUCTIONS

1. Melt butter over medium heat in a large skillet or pan (one that has a lid). Season chicken with salt and pepper to taste, and Italian seasoning.

2. Brown chicken in the butter for 1-2 minutes on each side. (Chicken shouldn't be cooked through at this point) Transfer chicken to a plate.

3. Add rice, chicken broth, lemon juice, and remaining Italian seasoning to the pan (no need to clean it first).

4. Place chicken on top, then cover and simmer over medium-low heat for 20-25 minutes until liquid is dissolved.

5. Garnish with fresh parsley or cilantro if desired and lemon wedges for squeezing.

6. Serve immediately.

One-pan lemon and chicken potato bake

Preparation time

1 hour 20 minutes

INGREDIENTS

- 2 garlic cloves, crushed

- 1cm piece fresh ginger, finely grated

- 1/2 teaspoon chilli powder (optional)

- 2 teaspoons fresh thyme leaves, plus extra to serve

- 1 tablespoon chopped fresh oregano leaves, plus extra to serve

- 1/3 cup Massel chicken style liquid stock

- 1/3 cup lemon juice

- 1/3 cup orange juice

- 500g baby red delight potatoes

- 1 brown onion, finely chopped

- 8 small chicken thigh cutlets (skin on), trimmed

- 1 teaspoon sweet paprika

- 1 small orange, sliced

- 1 lemon, sliced

- 1 tablespoon extra virgin olive oil

- 100g green beans, trimmed, cut into thirds

Instructions

1. Preheat oven to 200C/180C fan-forced.

2. Combine garlic, ginger, chilli powder (if using), thyme, oregano, stock, and lemon and orange juice in a jug.

3. Cut 2mm-thick slices into the top of each potato, being careful not to cut the whole way through.

4. Sprinkle onion over the base of a 25cm (12-cup-capacity) roasting pan.

5. Top with chicken. Arrange potatoes in between chicken pieces.

6. Pour stock mixture over chicken and potatoes.

7. Sprinkle with paprika.

8. Top with orange and lemon slices.

9. Drizzle with oil.

10. Season well with salt and pepper.

11. Bake for 50 minutes, basting with stock mixture during cooking.

12. Add beans, pushing into stock mixture.

13. Cook for a further 10 minutes or until chicken and potatoes are golden and cooked through.

14. Serve sprinkled with extra thyme and oregano.

Butter Chicken

Preparation time

1 hour 30 minutes

INGREDIENTS

- 1kg chicken thigh fillets, halved

- 1/3 cup raw cashews

- 1/4 cup ghee

- 1 brown onion, halved sliced

- 4 cardamom pods, bruised

- 1 cinnamon stick

- Pinch of ground cloves

- 410g can tomato puree

- 1 tablespoon white vinegar

- 3/4 cup thickened cream, plus extra to drizzle

- 4 cups steamed basmati rice, to serve

- 2 small pappadums, to serve

- Fresh coriander sprigs, to serve

MARINADE

- 1/2 cup plain Greek-style yoghurt

- 2 tablespoons tomato paste

- 3 garlic cloves, crushed

- 3cm piece fresh ginger, finely grated

- 2 teaspoons garam masala

- 2 teaspoons ground coriander

- 2 teaspoons ground cumin

- 3 teaspoons sweet paprika

- 1/2 teaspoon chilli powder

Instructions

1. Make Marinade: Combine yoghurt, tomato paste, garlic, ginger, garam masala, ground coriander, cumin, paprika and chilli powder in a large glass or ceramic bowl.

2. Add chicken to marinade, turning to coat. Cover.

3.   Refrigerate overnight to allow flavours to develop.

4.   Using a small food processor, process cashews with 1 tablespoon water until mixture forms a smooth paste, adding an extra tablespoon of water if needed.

5. Melt ghee in a large heavy-based saucepan over medium-high heat. Add onion. Cook, stirring, for 5 minutes or until softened.

6. Add chicken and marinade.

7. Cook, stirring, for 6 to 8 minutes or until chicken just starts to change colour. 5 Add cardamom, cinnamon, cloves and cashew paste.

8. Cook for 1 minute. Add tomato puree and vinegar. Season with salt and pepper.

9. Stir to combine.

10. Bring to the boil.

11. Reduce heat to low.

12. Cover. Simmer, stirring occasionally, for 1 hour or until chicken is tender and sauce has thickened. Stir in cream.

13. Serve butter chicken with rice and pappadums, drizzled with extra cream and sprinkled with coriander.

Chicken with tandoori cauliflower and herb sauce

Preparation time

1 hour

INGREDIENTS

- 2 tablespoons vegetable oil

- 2 garlic cloves, crushed

- 2cm piece fresh ginger, finely grated

- 2 tablespoons chopped fresh coriander leaves

- 4 large chicken thigh cutlets, skin on

- 2 tablespoons tandoori paste

- 1 tablespoon finely grated lemon rind

- 1 tablespoon honey

- 1 large (1kg) cauliflower, cut into thick wedges

- 200g plain Greek-style yoghurt

- 2 teaspoons lemon juice

- 1/2 cup fresh coriander leaves

- 1/2 cup fresh flat-leaf parsley leaves

- 200g green beans, trimmed

- 80g baby spinach

- 2 tablespoons natural flaked almonds, toasted

- 1 lemon, cut into wedges

Instructions

1. Preheat oven to 220C/200C fan-forced.

2. Line a large baking tray with baking paper.

3. Combine half the oil, garlic, ginger and chopped coriander in a bowl.

4. Trim excess fat from chicken.

5. Place chicken on prepared tray. Rub all over with oil mixture.

6. Roast, skin-side up, for 15 minutes.

7. Combine remaining oil, curry paste, lemon rind and honey in a large bowl.

8. Add cauliflower, rubbing with mixture to coat.

9. Place on tray with chicken.

10. Bake for a further 25 minutes or until cauliflower is golden and tender and chicken is cooked through.

11. Meanwhile, place yoghurt, lemon juice, 1/4 cup coriander leaves and 1/4 cup parsley in a small food processor.

12. Process until smooth and combined.

13. Cook beans in a medium saucepan of boiling water for 1 minute or until just tender. Drain. Refresh under cold water. Drain well.

14. Place beans, spinach, almonds and remaining coriander and parsley leaves in a bowl. Toss to combine.

15. Serve chicken and cauliflower with herb sauce, bean salad and lemon wedges.

Veal, sun-dried tomato and pine nut meatballs

Preparation time

30 minutes

INGREDIENTS

- 500g veal mince

- 3/4 cup fresh breadcrumbs

- 1 egg, lightly beaten

- 1/3 cup sun-dried tomatoes, finely chopped

- 2 tablespoons pine nuts, toasted

- 1 tablespoon fresh basil, finely chopped, plus extra leaves to serve

- 2 tablespoons extra virgin olive oil

CREAMY PESTO DIPPING SAUCE

- 1 cup fresh basil leaves, firmly packed

- 1 garlic clove, chopped

- 2 tablespoons parmesan, grated

- 1 tablespoon pine nuts, toasted

- 2 tablespoons extra virgin olive oil

- 1 tablespoon lemon juice

- 1/4 cup sour cream

Preparation time

1. Place mince, breadcrumbs, egg, tomato, pine nuts and basil in a bowl. Season with salt and pepper. Mix well. Roll level tablespoons of mince mixture into balls.

2. Heat oil in a large frying pan over medium-high heat. Cook meatballs, in batches, turning, for 5 to 7 minutes or until browned all over and cooked through. Drain on paper towel.

3. Meanwhile, make Creamy Pesto Dipping Sauce; Place basil, garlic, parmesan and pine nuts in a small food processor.

4. Process until finely chopped. With motor operating, gradually add oil and lemon juice until pesto is almost smooth.

5. Add sour cream.

6. Process until combined.

7. Serve meatballs with dipping sauce and extra basil leaves.

Slow-cooked beef pot roast with thyme gremolata

Preparation time

4 hours 40 minutes

INGREDIENTS

- 2kg piece beef chuck roast

- 2 tablespoons extra virgin olive oil

- 20g butter

- 1 large leek, trimmed, halved lengthways, thinly sliced

- 4 garlic cloves, crushed

- 4 sprigs fresh thyme

- 2 tablespoons plain flour

- 1 1/2 cups Massel beef stock

- 1 cup red wine

- 1/4 cup balsamic vinegar

- 800g small chat potatoes

- 2 bunches baby (Dutch) carrots, trimmed, peeled

THYME GREMOLATA

- 1/4 cup fresh flat-leaf parsley leaves, chopped

* 1 tablespoon fresh thyme leaves, roughly chopped

* 2 teaspoons lemon zest

Instructions

1. Place beef on a board.

2. Tie up with kitchen string at 3cm intervals to secure.

3. Heat 1/2 the oil in a large heavy-based, flameproof casserole dish over medium-high heat. Cook beef, turning, for 10 minutes or until browned all over.

4. Transfer to a plate.

5. Reduce heat to medium. Heat butter and remaining oil in dish.

6. Add leek. Cook, stirring, for 6 to 8 minutes or until leek has softened.

7. Add garlic and thyme.

8. Cook, stirring, for 1 minute or until fragrant.

9. Add flour. Cook, stirring, for 1 minute.

10. Gradually stir in stock, wine and vinegar.

11. Bring to the boil. Return beef to dish. Cover.

12. Reduce heat to low. Simmer for 3 hours, turning beef halfway through cooking.

13. Add potatoes.

14. Simmer, uncovered, for 30 minutes.

15. Add carrot.

16. Simmer, uncovered, for a further 30 minutes or until vegetables and meat are tender.

17. Meanwhile, make Thyme Gremolata; Combine parsley, thyme and lemon zest in a small bowl.

18. Transfer beef to a board. Discard string.

19. Shred beef into large pieces. Discard thyme sprigs from sauce.

20. Return beef to dish.

21. Serve beef with vegetable mixture and sprinkle with gremolata.

Sticky marmalade and apricot chicken

Preparation time

55 minutes

INGREDIENTS

• 8 small chicken thigh cutlets, with skin (see notes)

• 1/4 cup orange marmalade

• 1/2 cup apricot nectar

• 2 garlic cloves, crushed

• 2 small oranges, thinly sliced

• 4 sprigs fresh thyme sprigs

• 500g Kent pumpkin, unpeeled, cut into wedges, halved

- 1 tablespoon extra virgin olive oil

- 150g green beans, trimmed, halved

- Chopped fresh flat-leaf parsley leaves, to serve

Instructions

1. Preheat oven to 220C/200C fan-forced.

2. Place chicken, skin-side up, on a large baking tray with sides.

3. Place marmalade, apricot nectar and garlic in a jug.

4. Stir to combine.

5. Spoon over chicken. Season with salt and pepper.

6. Add orange slices and thyme to tray.

7. Roast for 20 minutes.

8. Add pumpkin to tray.

9. Drizzle with oil. Season with salt and pepper.

10. Roast for a further 25 minutes, or until chicken is cooked through, adding beans to the tray in the last 5 minutes of cooking.

11. Serve sprinkled with parsley (see notes).

Cider-poached salmon, grape and brown rice salad

Preparation time

35 minutes

INGREDIENTS

- 1 1/2 cups brown medium-grain rice

- 500ml apple cider

- 1 teaspoon whole black peppercorns

- 2 dried bay leaves

- 4cm piece fresh ginger, peeled, thickly sliced

- 3 sprigs fresh thyme

- 4 x 200g boneless salmon fillets, skin on

- 1 small Granny Smith apple, halved, cored, thinly sliced

- 2 baby fennel, trimmed, very thinly sliced (fronds reserved)

- 250g green seedless grapes, halved

- 2 tablespoons finely chopped fresh chives

* 80g baby rocket

DRESSING

* 1/2 cup apple cider vinegar

* 1/3 cup extra virgin olive oil

* 1 tablespoon chopped fresh dill

* 2 teaspoons wholegrain mustard

* Pinch of sugar

Instructions

1. Cook rice following packet directions. Refresh under cold water.

2. Drain well. Cool.

3. Meanwhile, place cider, 2 cups water, peppercorns, bay leaves, ginger and thyme in a large, deep frying pan over high heat.

4. Bring to the boil.

5. Reduce heat to low.

6. Add salmon.

7. Cover.

8. Simmer gently for 8 to 10 minutes, for medium, or until cooked to your liking.

9. Remove from heat.

10. Using a spatula, carefully lift salmon from liquid and transfer to a plate.

11. Discard poaching liquid.

12. Make Dressing: Whisk vinegar, oil, dill, mustard and sugar together in a jug.

13. Place apple, rice, fennel, grape and chives in a large bowl.

14. Drizzle with 1/2 the dressing.

15. Season well.

16. Toss to combine.

17. Arrange rice mixture and rocket on a serving plate.

18. Flake salmon, discarding skin, and place on top of rice.

19. Drizzle with remaining dressing. Sprinkle with reserved fennel fronds.

20. Serve.

Chilli tofu zoodles

Preparation time

15 minutes

INGREDIENTS

- 2 tablespoons chilli-infused extra virgin olive oil

- 300g firm tofu, cut into 1cm pieces

- 500g Coles Australian Zucchini Noodles* (see tip)

- 1 carrot, peeled, cut into long matchsticks

- 1 long red chilli, thinly sliced

Instructions

1. Heat half the oil in a large frying pan over medium-high heat.

2. Cook the tofu, turning occasionally, for 5 mins or until golden brown.

3. Transfer to a plate.

4. Add the zucchini to the pan and cook, tossing, for 2 mins or until just heated through.

5. Add the carrot and toss to combine.

6. Add the tofu to the zucchini mixture and toss to combine.

7. Sprinkle with the chilli and drizzle with the remaining oil. Season

One-pan summer-style chicken

Preparation time

1 hour 30 minutes

INGREDIENTS

- 2 tablespoons extra virgin olive oil

- 6 large chicken thigh cutlets, skin on, trimmed

- 1 brown onion, finely chopped

- 2 small carrots, finely chopped

- 2 celery stalks, finely chopped

- 1 red capsicum, finely chopped

- 1 large garlic clove, finely chopped

- 1 tablespoon coriander seeds

- 2 dried bay leaves

- 1/2 cup white wine vinegar

- 1/3 cup dry white wine

- 5 sprigs fresh thyme

- 1 tablespoon honey

- Steamed couscous, to serve

- Lemon wedges, to serve

- Fresh coriander, to serve

Instructions

1. Preheat oven to 200C/180C fan-forced.

2. Heat 1/2 the oil in a large, heavy-based flameproof casserole dish over medium- high heat.

3. Cook chicken for 5 minutes each side or until browned.

4. Transfer to a plate.

5. Heat remaining oil in pan over medium- high heat.

6. Cook onion, carrot, celery and capsicum, stirring occasionally, for 8 to 10 minutes or until vegetables are just tender.

7. Add garlic, coriander seeds and bay leaves.

8. Cook, stirring, for 1 minute or until fragrant.

9. Add vinegar, wine and 1/2 cup water.

10. Bring to a simmer.

11. Return chicken to pan.

12. Add thyme. Season. Cover.

13. Bake for 25 minutes.

14. Remove lid. Spoon over sauce mixture.

15. Drizzle with honey.

16. Bake for 25 minutes or until chicken is browned and cooked through.

17. Serve with couscous, lemon wedges and coriander sprigs.

Chicken Alfredo

Preparation time

15 minutes

INGREDIENTS

- 375g fettuccine

- 25g unsalted butter

- 1 eschalot, very finely chopped

- 3/4 cup Bulla Cooking Cream

- 1 cup finely grated parmesan (see notes), plus

extra to serve

- 1 cooked chicken breast fillet, shredded

- Shredded fresh flat-leaf parsley leaves, to serve

Instructions

1. Cook pasta in a large saucepan of boiling, salted water, following packet directions (see notes). Reserve 1 cup of cooking water. Drain pasta and set aside.

2. Meanwhile, melt butter in a large frying pan over medium-high heat.

3. Add eschalot. Cook, stirring, for 2 minutes or until soft. Add cream.

4. Bring to a simmer.

5. Reduce heat to medium-low.

6. Simmer for 3 minutes.

7. Remove from heat. Add parmesan. Stir until smooth.

8. Season with salt and pepper.

9. Increase heat to medium. Return pan to heat.

10. Add pasta, chicken and 1/2 the reserved pasta water.

11. Toss gently for 2 minutes or until the sauce thickens and coats the pasta (sauce should not be pooled in the bottom of the pan), adding more reserved pasta water, if needed.

12. Remove from heat.

13. Sprinkle with extra parmesan and parsley. Serve.

Creamy chicken and vegetable pasta bake

Preparation time

50 minutes

INGREDIENTS

- 375g dried fusilli pasta

- 1 1/2 cups small broccoli florets

- 1 cup frozen peas and corn

- 1 1/2 tablespoons light margarine

- 1/4 cup plain flour

- 2 1/2 cups warm reduced-fat milk

- 1 cup grated Devondale Tasty Cheese Block (500g)

- 3 cups chopped cooked chicken

- 100g baby spinach

- 2 green onions, thinly sliced

- 1/4 cup panko breadcrumbs

Instructions

1. Cook pasta in a large saucepan of boiling, salted water, following packet directions until tender, adding broccoli, and peas and corn in the last 2 minutes of cooking time. Drain well. Return pasta mixture to pan.

2. Meanwhile, melt margarine in a medium saucepan over medium heat. Add flour.

3. Cook, stirring, for 1 to 2 minutes or until mixture bubbles.

4. Gradually stir in warm milk. Bring to the boil.

5. Reduce heat to low.

6. Cook, stirring, for 4 to 5 minutes or until sauce thickens. Season with salt and pepper.

7. Stir in 1/4 cup cheese.

8. Preheat oven to 200C/180C fan-forced. Grease a 6cm-deep, 2.5-litre (10-cup-capacity) ovenproof dish.

9. Add sauce, chicken, spinach and onion to pasta.

10. Stir to combine. Spoon mixture into prepared dish.

11. Sprinkle with remaining cheese and breadcrumbs.

12. Bake for 15 to 20 minutes or until golden.

13. Stand for 5 minutes. Serve.

Portuguese chicken drumsticks and salad

Preparation time

45 minutes

INGREDIENTS

- 3/4 cup flat-leaf parsley leaves

- 1 long red chilli, finely chopped

- 1 teaspoon dried oregano

- 2 teaspoons brown sugar

- 2 garlic cloves, crushed

- 1 1/2 teaspoons smoked paprika

- 2 tablespoons olive oil

- 1/4 cup (60ml) apple cider vinegar

- 8 Coles RSPCA Approved Chicken Drumsticks

- Olive oil spray

- 4 small Red Royale potatoes

- 100g baby rocket leaves

- 250g cherry tomatoes, quartered

- 1/2 small red onion, thinly sliced

Instructions

1. Finely chop 2 tablespoons of the parsley and place in a large bowl.

2. Add the chilli, oregano, sugar, garlic, 1 teaspoon of the paprika, 2 teaspoons of the oil and 1 tablespoon of the vinegar. Stir to combine.

3. Use a large sharp knife to cut 3 slits in each chicken drumstick.

4. Add to marinade and toss to coat. Set aside for 15 mins to marinate.

5. Spray a barbecue grill or chargrill with oil and heat on medium.

6. Cook chicken, turning occasionally, for 10-12 mins or until cooked through.

7. Meanwhile, place potatoes on a microwave-safe plate lined with paper towel. Sprinkle with water.

8. Cover with paper towel.

9. Microwave on high for 4-5 mins or until just tender.

10. Thickly slice and place in a bowl with remaining paprika and 2 teaspoons of the remaining oil. Toss to coat.

11. Cook potato with chicken for 2-3 mins each side or until golden.

12. Place the rocket, tomato, onion and the remaining parsley, oil and vinegar in a bowl and toss to combine. Season.

13.   Add potato and gently toss to combine.

Arrange on a serving platter and top with the

chicken.

Quinoa-crumbed veal schnitzel with shaved fennel and apple salad

Preparation time

35 minutes

INGREDIENTS

- 1/2 cup rice flour

- 1/3 cup milk

- 1 egg

- 1 1/2 cups quinoa flakes

- 2 tablespoons finely chopped fresh chives

- 2 teaspoons finely grated lemon rind

- 4 x 125g veal schnitzels (uncrumbed)

- 1 fennel, fronds reserved

- 2 small pink lady apples

- 2 cups watercress sprigs

- 2 tablespoons lemon juice

- 1 tablespoon extra virgin olive oil

- 1 teaspoon wholegrain mustard

- Vegetable oil, for shallow-frying

- Lemon wedges, to serve

Instructions

1. Place rice flour on a plate.

2. Season with salt and pepper. Whisk milk and egg in a shallow bowl until combined.

3. Combine quinoa, chives and lemon rind on a plate.

4. Toss 1 piece veal schnitzel in rice flour mixture, shaking off excess. Dip in egg mixture. Coat in quinoa mixture, pressing down firmly.

5. Place on a tray. Repeat with remaining veal, rice flour, egg and quinoa mixtures. Refrigerate for 10 minutes (see notes).

6. Meanwhile, using a mandolin or sharp knife, thinly shave fennel. Halve and core apples. Cut into thin wedges.

7. Combine fennel, reserved fennel fronds, apple and watercress in a medium bowl.

8. Whisk lemon juice, oil and mustard in a small bowl to combine. Season with salt and pepper.

9. Add dressing to fennel mixture. Toss to combine.

10. Pour enough oil into a large frying pan to come 5mm up side of pan. Heat over medium-high heat.

11. Cook schnitzels for 2 minutes each side or until just cooked through. Drain on paper towel.

12. Serve schnitzels with fennel and apple salad and lemon wedges.

Chicken with confit potatoes and glazed carrots

Preparation time

50 minutes

INGREDIENTS

- 300g kipfler potatoes, peeled, halved lengthways

- Extra virgin olive oil, to confit

- 4 large carrots, halved, quartered lengthways

- 2 tablespoons extra virgin olive oil, extra

- 1 tablespoon brown sugar

- 4 small (200g each) chicken breast fillets (skin on)

- 3/4 cup dry white wine

Instructions

1. Place potato in a medium saucepan. Add enough oil to just cover potato. Place saucepan over low heat.

2. Cook for 45 minutes (do not allow oil to bubble) or until tender.

3. Remove pan from heat.

4. Cover to keep warm.

5. Meanwhile, place carrot, 1/2 the extra oil, brown sugar and 1/2 cup water in a medium frying pan over medium-high heat.

6. Bring to a simmer. Reduce heat to medium.

7. Cook, turning once or twice, for 15 minutes or until carrot is just tender and caramelised, and liquid has evaporated.

8. Using a meat mallet or rolling pin, pound chicken until 1.5cm-thick. Season both sides of chicken with salt and pepper.

9. Using a small knife, prick the chicken skin all over about 10 times

10. Place remaining extra oil in a large frying pan.

11. Place chicken in pan, skin-side down, and top with a heavy saucepan to weigh down the chicken during cooking.

12. Place over medium heat.

13. Cook for 10 minutes or until skin is deep golden brown and very crisp. Remove saucepan. Turn chicken.

14. Cook for a further 4 minutes or until just cooked through. Transfer to a plate.

15. Cover loosely with foil to keep warm.

16. Return frying pan to heat. Add wine. Bring to a simmer.

17. Cook, stirring to lift any cooked-on bits from the bottom of the pan, for 2 minutes or until reduced by half. Season with salt and pepper.

18. Spoon sauce onto each serving plate (see note).

19. Using a slotted spoon, transfer potato to plates.

20. Top with carrot and chicken. Serve
immediately.